# THE

# MEDITERRANEAN

# DIET COOKBOOK

# FOR BEGINNERS

## 2024

## BY GENEVA J. SPOON

# Contents

7.     Chicken and vegetable soup with whole wheat roll:

8.     Tuna salad sandwich on whole wheat bread with lettuce, tomato, and mayo:

9.     Vegetable lasagna with ricotta cheese, tomato sauce, and spinach:

10.     Quinoa salad with chickpeas, tomatoes, cucumbers, parsley, lemon juice, and olive oil:

11.     Minestrone soup with parmesan cheese and whole wheat breadstick:

12.     Roasted vegetable sandwich on whole wheat bread with hummus,

13.     Nicoise salad with tuna, hard-boiled eggs, potatoes, green beans, olives, and vinaigrette dressing

SNACKS

1.     Hummus with carrot and celery sticks is a simple and healthy snack that you can make at home.

2.     Greek yogurt with honey and walnuts

3.     Orange Almond Cake:

4.     Roasted chickpeas

5.     Greek yogurt dip with fresh veggies

6.     Mediterranean pinwheels

7.     Dried figs and pistachios

8.     Celery sticks with cream cheese

DINNER

1.     Baked salmon with lemon and herbs, roasted asparagus, and brown rice:

2.     Vegetable and cheese frittata with whole wheat

3.     Spaghetti with tomato and basil sauce, green salad, and garlic bread

4.     Shrimp and vegetable stir-fry with brown rice

5.     Lamb chops with mint sauce, couscous, and roasted carrots

6.     Ratatouille (vegetable stew) with crusty bread

7.     Roasted pork loin with apple sauce, mashed potatoes, and broccoli

8.     Fish tacos with cabbage slaw, avocado, salsa, and sour cream:

9.     Mushroom risotto with parmesan cheese, green salad

10.      Moroccan tagine (stew) with lamb, chickpeas, apricots, and almonds, couscous

11.      Paella (rice dish) with shrimp, chicken, sausage, and peas:

CHAPTER 5: TIPS AND TRICKS FOR STICKING TO THE MEDITERRANEAN DIET: how to eat out, travel, and deal with cravings

CHAPTER 6: FAQS ON MEDITERRANEAN DIET

CONCLUSION

# INTRODUCTION

Hi! Welcome to this amazing book on Mediterranean diet. I know you might have heard about it and might have been wondering what it's all about. Alright let's get into it.

The traditional eating practices of people who reside in nations like Greece, Italy, France, and Spain, which are located around the Mediterranean Sea, are the inspiration for the Mediterranean diet. It is based on plant-based foods, including fresh produce, whole grains, legumes, nuts, seeds, and spices. There is a moderate amount of meat and saturated fat, as well as moderate amounts of fish, seafood, dairy, poultry, and eggs. The primary source of additional fat is olive oil.

The Mediterranean diet has been demonstrated to improve both mental and physical function in older persons and to lower the risk of heart disease, metabolic syndrome, diabetes, some malignancies, and depression.

Here are some simple adjustments you can make to your daily routine to integrate this healthy diet:

- Replace any current fats with extra virgin olive oil.

- Replace packaged snacks with a handful of raw nuts every day for a healthy alternative.

- Include whole grains in the meal, such as whole grain bread.

- Add a salad to the start or conclusion of each meal.

- Expand the selection of veggies on the menu.

- Consume three or more servings of legumes every week.

Consume less meat. Choose moderate quantities of lean poultry. Red meat should only be consumed seldom.

- Increase your weekly intake of fish to two to three servings.

- Wine can be substituted for other alcoholic beverages in moderation.

- Avoid sugary drinks. Use water in place of soda and juice.

Eat fewer desserts that are heavy in sugar and fat. The best fruit is fresh or poached.

The Mediterranean diet is not just about food but also about an active lifestyle that includes plenty of exercise and enjoying meals with family and friends. It's not only about what we eat but also how we eat. Enjoying delicious food with good company is a big part of the Mediterranean lifestyle!

The Mediterranean diet is a way of eating that is inspired by the traditional foods and cuisines of the countries bordering the Mediterranean Sea. It is not a strict diet plan, but rather a general pattern of eating that emphasizes whole, minimally processed foods, mostly plants, healthy fats, and a variety of flavors.

# CHAPTER ONE: BENEFITS OF THE MEDITERRANEAN DIET

The Mediterranean diet has many health benefits. Some of the benefits are:

- It can reduce your risk of heart disease by lowering your blood pressure, cholesterol, and inflammation.

- It can slow down worsening memory loss and prevent Alzheimer's disease by improving your brain function and blood flow.

- It can help you lose weight and maintain a healthy body mass index (BMI) by increasing your metabolism and satiety.

- It can reduce your risk of having a stroke by preventing blood clots and improving your blood vessel health.

- It can help you prevent or manage type 2 diabetes by regulating your blood sugar and insulin levels.

**To follow the Mediterranean diet, you can make some simple changes to your eating habits, such as:**

- Make vegetables the main part of your dish and eat more fruits as snacks or desserts.

- Go meatless at least once a week and choose fish and seafood twice a week as your protein sources.

- Eat some dairy products, such as plain Greek yogurt and cheese, in moderation.

- Switch to whole grains, such as barley, brown rice, and oats, instead of refined grains, such as white bread and pasta.

- Use olive oil as your msain cooking fat and limit butter and other animal fats.

- Season your food with herbs and spices instead of salt and sugar.

- Enjoy red wine in moderation (optional) and drink plenty of water.

- Be physically active and socialize with your friends and family.

The Mediterranean diet is not only good for your health, but also for your taste buds. It offers a variety of delicious dishes that are easy to prepare and enjoy. You can find some recipes and meal plans on the web or in books. I hope this helps you learn more about the Mediterranean diet and why it is good for you.

**CHAPTER TWO: BASICS OF THE MEDITERRANEAN DIET**

The basics of the Mediterranean diet are:

- It is a way of eating that is inspired by the traditional foods and cuisines of the countries bordering the Mediterranean Sea, such as France, Spain, Greece, and Italy.

- It emphasizes whole, minimally processed foods, mostly plants, healthy fats, and a variety of flavors.

- It has many health benefits, such as reducing the risk of heart disease, diabetes, stroke, cognitive decline, and premature death.

There are some foods that is recommended to be eaten on the Mediterranean diet they are:

- Vegetables: tomatoes, broccoli, kale, spinach, onions, cauliflower, carrots, Brussels sprouts, cucumbers, potatoes, sweet potatoes, turnips

- Fruits: apples, bananas, oranges, grapes, pears, peaches, melons, berries

- Whole grains: barley, brown rice, oats, quinoa, bulgur, farro, couscous

- Legumes: beans, lentils, chickpeas, peas

- Nuts and seeds: almonds, walnuts, pistachios, cashews, sunflower seeds, pumpkin seeds

- Healthy fats: olive oil, avocado oil

- Fish and seafood: salmon, tuna, sardines, mackerel, shrimp

- Dairy products: cheese (especially feta), yogurt (especially Greek), milk

- Eggs: boiled or poached eggs

- Herbs and spices: basil, oregano, parsley, rosemary, thyme

Some of the foods to limit or avoid on the Mediterranean diet are:

- Processed foods: chips, crackers, cookies

- Added sugars: candy, soda

- Refined grains: white bread, white pasta

- Red meat: beef, pork

- Processed meat: bacon, sausage

- Other animal fats: butter, lard

- Salt and sugar: use herbs and spices instead to flavor your food

Now let's look at some tips on how to follow the Mediterranean diet are:

- Make vegetables the main part of your dish and eat more fruits as snacks or desserts.

- Go meatless at least once a week and choose fish and seafood twice a week as your protein sources.

- Eat some dairy products in moderation and switch to whole grains instead of refined grains.

- Use olive oil as your main cooking fat and limit butter and other animal fats.

- Season your food with herbs and spices instead of salt and sugar.

- Enjoy red wine in moderation (optional) and drink plenty of water.

- Be physically active and socialize with your friends and family.

# CHAPTER THREE: THE MEDITERRANEAN LIFESTYLE

The Mediterranean lifestyle is more than just a diet. It is also a way of living that involves physical activity, social interaction, and mindfulness. Here are some tips on how you can incorporate these aspects into your daily routine:

-Physical exercise: The Mediterranean way of life promotes outdoor recreation and physical activity. You don't have to visit the gym or adhere to a rigid exercise schedule. Simply add additional physical activity to your regular routine by walking, riding, gardening, dancing, or playing with your children or animals. Aim for 150 minutes or more of moderate-intensity exercise each week.

- Social interaction: The Mediterranean way of life also places a high priority on ties to the local community. Spending quality time with them, eating meals together, commemorating special milestones, and offering support to one another will help you develop meaningful relationships with your family, friends, neighbors, and coworkers. Strong social bonds have been linked to longer lifespans and better physical and mental health, according to studies.

- Mindfulness: Adopting a Mediterranean lifestyle encourages you to pay attention to your emotions, body, and food. By chewing each bite thoroughly, paying attention to your hunger and fullness cues, and selecting nourishing and enjoyable foods, you can practice mindfulness. Additionally, you can develop mindfulness by meditating, taking deep breaths, expressing your thanks, or partaking in enjoyable and relaxing activities.

By following these tips, you can embrace the Mediterranean lifestyle and enjoy its benefits for your health and well-being.

# CHAPTER FOUR: MEAL PLANS AND RECIPES (A 14-Day meal plan)

A 14-day meal plan for the Mediterranean diet is a great way to enjoy the delicious and healthy foods of this eating pattern. Here is a sample meal plan that you can use as a guide, but feel free to adjust it according to your preferences and needs. You can also find more recipes and tips on the web or in books.

Day 1

- Breakfast: Greek yogurt with fresh berries and granola

- Lunch: Lentil and vegetable soup with whole wheat bread

- Snack: Hummus with carrot and celery sticks

- Dinner: Baked salmon with lemon and herbs, roasted asparagus, and brown rice

Day 2

- Breakfast: Oatmeal with sliced almonds and dried apricots

- Lunch: Mediterranean salad with lettuce, tomatoes, cucumbers, olives, feta cheese, and grilled chicken

- Snack: Apple slices with peanut butter

- Dinner: Vegetable and cheese frittata with whole wheat toast


Day 3

- Breakfast: Whole wheat pancakes with fresh strawberries and maple syrup

- Lunch: Turkey and cheese sandwich on whole wheat bread with lettuce, tomato, and mustard

- Snack: Greek yogurt with honey and walnuts

- Dinner: Spaghetti with tomato and basil sauce, green salad, and garlic bread

Day 4

- Breakfast: Scrambled eggs with spinach and cheese, whole wheat pita bread

- Lunch: Vegetable and bean chili with tortilla chips and salsa

- Snack: Orange and almond cake

- Dinner: Roasted chicken with rosemary and lemon, roasted potatoes, and green beans


Day 5

- Breakfast: Smoothie with banana, spinach, milk, and flax seeds

- Lunch: Tomato and mozzarella salad with balsamic dressing, whole wheat crackers, and grapes

- Snack: Cheese and crackers

- Dinner: Shrimp and vegetable stir-fry with brown rice

Day 6

- Breakfast: French toast with fresh blueberries and whipped cream

- Lunch: Vegetable and cheese pizza on whole wheat crust

- Snack: Trail mix with nuts, dried fruits, and dark chocolate chips

- Dinner: Lamb chops with mint sauce, couscous, and roasted carrots


Day 7

- Breakfast: Granola bar and a glass of orange juice

- Lunch: Chicken and vegetable soup with whole wheat roll

- Snack: Fresh fruit salad

- Dinner: Ratatouille (vegetable stew) with crusty bread

Day 8

- Breakfast: Omelet with mushrooms, cheese, and ham, whole wheat toast

- Lunch: Tuna salad sandwich on whole wheat bread with lettuce, tomato, and mayo

- Snack: Popcorn

- Dinner: Beef and vegetable kebabs with tzatziki sauce (yogurt, cucumber, garlic), pita bread, and Greek salad


Day 9

- Breakfast: Cereal with milk and sliced banana

- Lunch: Vegetable lasagna with ricotta cheese, tomato sauce, and spinach

- Snack: Chocolate chip cookies

- Dinner: Roasted pork loin with apple sauce, mashed potatoes, and broccoli


Day 10

- Breakfast: Muffin and a cup of coffee or tea

- Lunch: Quinoa salad with chickpeas, tomatoes, cucumbers, parsley, lemon juice, and olive oil

- Snack: Dried figs and pistachios

- Dinner: Fish tacos with cabbage slaw, avocado, salsa, and sour cream


Day 11

- Breakfast: Waffles with fresh raspberries and whipped cream

- Lunch: Minestrone soup with parmesan cheese and whole wheat breadstick

- Snack: Celery sticks with cream cheese and raisins

- Dinner: Chicken curry with coconut milk, cauliflower rice, and naan bread

Day 12

- Breakfast: Egg muffins with cheese, bacon, and spinach

- Lunch: Greek wrap with grilled chicken, lettuce, tomato, cucumber, olives, feta cheese, and tzatziki sauce

- Snack: Banana bread

- Dinner: Mushroom risotto with parmesan cheese, green salad

Day 13

- Breakfast: Smoothie bowl with frozen berries, yogurt, granola, and chia seeds

- Lunch: Roasted vegetable sandwich on whole wheat bread with

hummus

- Snack: Date balls

- Dinner: Moroccan tagine (stew) with lamb, chickpeas, apricots

,and almonds ,couscous


Day 14

-Breakfast : Croissant and a glass of milk

-Lunch : Nicoise salad with tuna ,hard-boiled eggs ,potatoes

,green beans ,olives ,and vinaigrette dressing

-Snack : Dark chocolate

-Dinner : Paella (rice dish)with shrimp ,chicken ,sausage ,and peas


I hope this meal plan helps you enjoy the Mediterranean diet and

its benefits. Now lets get into the recipes

# BREAKFAST

## 1. Greek yogurt with fresh berries and granola

- Ingredients:

    - 1 cup of plain Greek yogurt

    - 1/4 teaspoon of vanilla extract (optional)

    - 1 cup of fresh berries (such as strawberries, blueberries, raspberries, or blackberries)

    - 1/2 cup of granola (such as oats and honey or oats and dark chocolate)

    - 1 tablespoon of honey (or to taste)

- Directions:

    - In a small bowl, stir the vanilla extract into the Greek yogurt if using.

- In a large glass or jar, layer half of the yogurt, half of the berries, and half of the granola. Repeat with the remaining yogurt, berries, and granola.

- Drizzle the honey over the top of the parfait.

- Enjoy your delicious and nutritious breakfast or snack!

## 2. oatmeal with sliced almonds and dried apricots

- Ingredients:

- 1 cup of rolled oats

- 2 cups of water or almond milk

- A pinch of salt

- 1/4 cup of sliced almonds

- 1/4 cup of chopped dried apricots

- 2 tablespoons of maple syrup or honey

- 1/2 teaspoon of vanilla extract (optional)

- Directions:

- In a medium saucepan, bring the water or almond milk and salt to a boil over high heat.

- Add the oats and reduce the heat to medium-low. Simmer, stirring occasionally, until the oats are soft and creamy, about 15 to 20 minutes.

- Stir in the almonds, apricots, maple syrup or honey, and vanilla extract if using.

- Enjoy your warm and hearty breakfast

3. **Whole wheat pancakes with fresh strawberries and maple syrup:**

- Ingredients:

    - 1 cup of whole wheat flour

    - 2 teaspoons of baking powder

    - 1/4 teaspoon of salt

    - 1/4 teaspoon of cinnamon

    - 1 cup of plain Greek yogurt

    - 3/4 cup of milk

    - 2 large eggs

    - 2 tablespoons of pure maple syrup

    - 1 teaspoon of vanilla extract

    - 2 tablespoons of coconut oil, melted and cooled slightly

    - Fresh strawberries, sliced, for serving

    - More maple syrup, for serving

- Directions:

- In a large bowl, whisk together the flour, baking powder, salt, and cinnamon.

- In a medium bowl, whisk together the yogurt, milk, eggs, maple syrup, and vanilla extract until well combined.

- Add the wet ingredients to the dry ingredients and stir gently until just combined. Do not over mix. Fold in the melted coconut oil.

- Heat a lightly greased griddle or skillet over medium-high heat. Drop about 1/4 cup of batter onto the griddle for each pancake. Cook until bubbles appear on the surface, about 3 minutes. Flip and cook until golden on the other side, about 2 more minutes. Repeat with the remaining batter, adding more oil or butter to the griddle as needed.

- Serve the pancakes hot with fresh strawberries and more maple syrup.

## 4. Scrambled eggs with spinach and cheese, whole wheat pita bread

- Ingredients:

  - 4 large eggs

  - 1/4 cup of milk

  - Salt and pepper to taste

  - 1 tablespoon of butter or oil

  - 2 cups of fresh spinach, washed and chopped

  - 1/4 cup of shredded cheddar cheese

  - 2 whole wheat pita breads, cut in half

- Directions:

  - In a medium bowl, whisk the eggs, milk, salt, and pepper until well combined.

- In a large skillet over medium-high heat, melt the butter or heat the oil. Add the spinach and cook, stirring occasionally, until wilted, about 5 minutes.

- Reduce the heat to medium-low and pour the egg mixture over the spinach. Cook, stirring gently, until the eggs are set, about 10 minutes.

- Sprinkle the cheese over the eggs and spinach and let it melt slightly.

- Warm the pita breads in a toaster oven or microwave if desired.

- Spoon the egg mixture into the pita halves and enjoy!

## 5.  Smoothie with banana, spinach, milk and flax seeds

- Ingredients:

- 1 ripe banana, peeled and frozen

- 1 cup of fresh spinach leaves, washed and stemmed

- 1 cup of milk of your choice (dairy or non-dairy)

- 1 tablespoon of flax seeds

- Directions:

- Add all the ingredients to a blender and blend on high speed until smooth and creamy. You may need to scrape down the sides of the blender or add more milk if the mixture is too thick.

- Pour the smoothie into a glass and enjoy!

## 6. French toast with fresh blueberries and whipped cream

- Ingredients:

- 4 large eggs

- 1 cup of milk

- 1/4 teaspoon of salt

- 1/4 teaspoon of cinnamon

- 8 slices of thick bread (such as brioche or challah)

- 2 tablespoons of butter or oil

- 2 cups of fresh blueberries

- 1/4 cup of maple syrup

- Whipped cream for serving

- Directions:

- In a shallow bowl, whisk together the eggs, milk, salt, and cinnamon until well combined.

- Dip each slice of bread into the egg mixture, turning to coat both sides. Let the excess drip off and place on a large plate.

- Heat a large skillet over medium-high heat and add some butter or oil. Cook the bread slices in batches until golden and crisp on both sides, about 3 minutes per side. Transfer to a serving platter and keep warm in a low oven if needed.

- In a small saucepan over medium heat, bring the blueberries and maple syrup to a boil. Reduce the heat and simmer until the blueberries are soft and the syrup is slightly thickened, about 10 minutes.

- Serve the French toast with the blueberry syrup and whipped cream on top.

**7. granola bar and a glass of orange juice is:**

- For the granola bar, you will need the following ingredients:

  - 1 cup of pitted dates

  - 2 cups of walnuts or Brazil nuts

  - 2 cups of desiccated coconut

- 3/4 cup of dried cranberries

- 3 tablespoons of water

- For the orange juice, you will need the following ingredients:

- 4 large oranges

- A juicer or a blender and a strainer

- To make the granola bar, follow these steps:

- First toast the walnuts slightly in an oven heated to 170 degrees Celsius. Let them cool down before adding them to your food processor along with dates, desiccated coconut and cranberries. Process until the mixture is well combined and has a crumbly texture.

- Now add gradually the water, a tablespoon at a time and keep processing until the mixture is sticky and holds together.

- Transfer the mixture to a baking dish lined with parchment paper and press it firmly into an even layer. Refrigerate for at least an hour or until firm.

   - Cut into bars and enjoy!


- To make the orange juice, follow these steps:

   - Wash and peel the oranges and cut them into quarters.

   - If you have a juicer, simply feed the orange pieces through the juicer and collect the juice in a pitcher or a glass. If you have a blender, blend the orange pieces until smooth and then strain the juice through a fine-mesh sieve or a cheesecloth.

   - Enjoy your fresh and refreshing orange juice!

## 8. Omelet with mushrooms, cheese and ham, and whole wheat toast:

- Ingredients:

  - 3 eggs

  - 2 tablespoons of milk

  - Salt and pepper to taste

  - 1 tablespoon of butter or oil

  - 1/4 cup of sliced mushrooms

  - 1/4 cup of diced ham

  - 1/4 cup of shredded cheese (such as cheddar or Swiss)

  - 2 slices of whole wheat bread

  - Optional: butter, jam, or honey for toast

- **Directions:**

- In a small bowl, whisk the eggs, milk, salt, and pepper until well combined.

- In a medium skillet over medium-high heat, heat the butter or oil and cook the mushrooms and ham until browned, stirring occasionally, for about 10 minutes. Transfer to a plate and keep warm.

- In the same skillet over medium-low heat, pour the egg mixture and swirl to cover the bottom of the pan. Cook until the eggs are almost set, about 5 minutes, lifting the edges with a spatula and tilting the pan to let the uncooked egg run underneath.

- Sprinkle the cheese over half of the omelet and top with the mushroom and ham mixture. Fold the other half of the omelet over the filling and slide onto a serving plate.

- Toast the bread in a toaster or oven until golden and crisp. Spread with butter, jam, or honey if desired.

- Enjoy your omelet with whole wheat toast!

**9. muffin with a cup of coffee or tea:**

- For the muffin, you will need the following ingredients:

    - 2 cups of all-purpose flour

    - 3 teaspoons of baking powder

    - 1/2 teaspoon of salt

    - 3/4 cup of white sugar

    - 1 egg

    - 1 cup of milk

    - 1/4 cup of vegetable oil

- For the coffee or tea, you will need the following ingredients:

    - Your preferred coffee beans or tea leaves

    - Water

- A coffee maker or a kettle and a teapot

- Optional: milk, cream, sugar, honey, or other sweeteners and flavorings


- To make the muffin, follow these steps:

- Preheat the oven to 400 degrees F (200 degrees C).

- In a large bowl, whisk together the flour, baking powder, salt, and sugar.

- In a small bowl, whisk together the egg, milk, and oil.

- Add the wet ingredients to the dry ingredients and stir gently until just combined. Do not overmix.

- Spoon the batter into greased or paper-lined muffin cups, filling them about two-thirds full.

- Bake for 20 to 25 minutes or until golden and a toothpick inserted in the center comes out clean.

- Let the muffins cool slightly before removing from the pan.

- To make the coffee or tea, follow these steps:

- For coffee, grind your coffee beans to your desired coarseness and measure out the amount you need according to your coffee maker's instructions. Fill the water reservoir with filtered water and turn on the machine. Wait until the coffee is brewed and pour into a mug. Add milk, cream, sugar, or other flavorings as desired.

- For tea, boil some water in a kettle and place your tea leaves in a teapot. Pour the hot water over the tea leaves and let them steep for 3 to 5 minutes or longer depending on your preference. Strain the tea into a cup and add milk, honey, or other sweeteners as desired.

Enjoy your muffin with a cup of coffee or tea!

## 10.Waffles with fresh raspberries and whipped cream:

- Ingredients:

    - 2 cups of all-purpose flour

    - 3 teaspoons of baking powder

    - 1/2 teaspoon of salt

    - 3/4 cup of white sugar

    - 1 egg

    - 1 cup of milk

    - 1/4 cup of vegetable oil

    - 2 cups of fresh raspberries

    - 1/4 cup of maple syrup

    - Whipped cream for serving

- Directions:

- In a large bowl, whisk together the flour, baking powder, salt, and sugar.

- In a small bowl, whisk together the egg, milk, and oil.

- Add the wet ingredients to the dry ingredients and stir gently until just combined. Do not overmix.

- Preheat a waffle iron and spray it with cooking spray. Spoon about 1/4 cup of batter onto the waffle iron and cook until golden and crisp, about 3 to 4 minutes. Repeat with the remaining batter.

- In a small saucepan over medium heat, bring the raspberries and maple syrup to a boil. Reduce the heat and simmer until the raspberries are soft and the syrup is slightly thickened, about 10 minutes.

- Serve the waffles with the raspberry syrup and whipped cream on top.

## 11.egg muffins with cheese, bacon, and spinach:

- Ingredients:

  - 6 eggs

  - 1/4 cup of milk

  - Salt and pepper to taste

  - 1/4 cup of shredded cheese (such as cheddar or Swiss)

  - 2 cups of fresh spinach, washed and chopped

  - 6 slices of bacon, cooked, drained of fat, and chopped

- Directions:

  - Preheat the oven to 350 degrees F and spray a 12-cup muffin pan with cooking spray.

  - In a medium bowl, whisk the eggs, milk, salt, and pepper until well combined.

  - Stir in the cheese, spinach, and bacon.

- Divide the mixture evenly among the muffin cups, filling them about 3/4 full.

- Bake for 20 to 25 minutes or until the eggs are set and golden.

- Let the muffins cool slightly before removing them from the pan.

- Enjoy your egg muffins with some toast or fruit if desired.

## 12.Croissant with a glass of milk

- For the croissant, you will need the following ingredients:

- 2 cups of all-purpose flour

- 3 teaspoons of baking powder

- 1/2 teaspoon of salt

- 3/4 cup of white sugar

- 1 egg

- 1 cup of milk

- 1/4 cup of vegetable oil

- 2/3 cup of unsalted butter, chilled

- For the milk, you will need the following ingredient:

- 1 cup of milk of your choice (dairy or non-dairy)

- To make the croissant, follow these steps:

- In a small bowl, combine the warm water, yeast, and 1 teaspoon of sugar. Let it stand until the yeast is foamy, about 5 minutes.

- In a large bowl, whisk together the flour, baking powder, salt, and sugar.

- In a medium bowl, whisk together the egg, milk, and oil.

- Add the wet ingredients to the dry ingredients and stir until a soft dough forms. Knead the dough on a lightly floured surface for about 10 minutes, until smooth and elastic. Place the dough in a lightly greased bowl, cover with plastic wrap, and refrigerate for at least 2 hours or overnight.

- Place the butter between two sheets of parchment paper and pound it with a rolling pin until it forms a rectangle about 8 x 5 inches. Refrigerate the butter until firm, about 30 minutes.

- On a lightly floured surface, roll out the dough into a rectangle about 16 x 10 inches. Place the butter in the center of the dough and fold the dough over it like a letter. Seal the edges and refrigerate for 30 minutes.

- Repeat the rolling and folding process two more times, chilling the dough for 30 minutes between each fold. Wrap the dough in plastic wrap and refrigerate for at least 4 hours or overnight.

- Preheat the oven to 375°F and line two baking sheets with parchment paper.

- On a lightly floured surface, roll out the dough into a rectangle about 20 x 12 inches. Cut the dough into triangles with two equal sides, about 5 inches long each. Stretch each triangle slightly and roll it up from the base to the tip. Place the croissants on the prepared baking sheets, curving them slightly. Cover them with a damp cloth and let them rise for about an hour, until puffy.

- In a small bowl, whisk together an egg and a tablespoon of water. Brush the egg wash over the croissants and bake them for 15 to 20 minutes, until golden and flaky.

- To make the milk, follow these steps:

- Pour the milk into a microwave-safe mug or glass and heat it in the microwave for about a minute, or until warm but not boiling. Alternatively, you can heat the milk in a small saucepan over low heat, stirring occasionally, until warm but not boiling.

- Enjoy your croissant with a glass of milk!

# LUNCH

**1. lentil and vegetable soup with whole wheat bread:**

- Ingredients:

  - 1 tablespoon of extra virgin olive oil

  - 1 onion, chopped

  - 2 carrots, peeled and diced

  - 2 celery stalks, sliced

  - 2 garlic cloves, minced

  - 1 teaspoon of dried thyme

  - 1 teaspoon of dried rosemary

  - 4 cups of vegetable broth

  - 2 cups of water

  - 1 cup of brown or green lentils, rinsed and drained

- 1 bay leaf

- Salt and pepper to taste

- 2 cups of baby spinach leaves

- 2 tablespoons of lemon juice

- Whole wheat bread, sliced and toasted, for serving

- Directions:

- In a large pot over medium-high heat, heat the oil and sauté the onion, carrot, celery, garlic, thyme, and rosemary for about 15 minutes, stirring occasionally, until the vegetables are soft and golden.

- Add the broth, water, lentils, bay leaf, salt, and pepper and bring to a boil. Reduce the heat and simmer, covered, for about 30 minutes or until the lentils are tender.

- Stir in the spinach and lemon juice and cook for another 5 minutes until the spinach is wilted.

- Discard the bay leaf and ladle the soup into bowls. Serve with whole wheat bread on the side.

## 2. Mediterranean salad with lettuce, tomatoes, cucumbers, olives, feta cheese, and grilled chicken:

- Ingredients:

   - 4 cups of chopped romaine lettuce

   - 2 cups of cherry tomatoes, halved

   - 1 large cucumber, peeled and diced

   - 1/4 cup of sliced black olives

   - 1/4 cup of crumbled feta cheese

   - 2 grilled chicken breasts, sliced

- For the dressing:

   - 1/4 cup of extra virgin olive oil

- 3 tablespoons of red wine vinegar

- 1 teaspoon of dried oregano

- 1/2 teaspoon of garlic powder

- Salt and pepper to taste

- Directions:

- In a large salad bowl, toss the lettuce, tomatoes, cucumber, olives, and feta cheese together.

- In a small jar with a tight-fitting lid, shake the olive oil, vinegar, oregano, garlic powder, salt, and pepper until well combined.

- Drizzle the dressing over the salad and toss to coat.

- Top the salad with the grilled chicken slices and serve.

3.  **A turkey and cheese sandwich on whole wheat bread with lettuce, tomato and mustard:**

- Ingredients:

  - 2 slices of whole wheat bread

  - 2 teaspoons of Dijon-style prepared mustard

  - 3 slices of smoked turkey breast

  - 1 slice of Colby-Monterey Jack cheese

  - 1 lettuce leaf

  - 2 tomato slices

- Directions:

  - Spread the mustard evenly on one side of each bread slice.

  - Layer the turkcy, cheese, lettuce, and tomato on one bread slice, mustard side up.

  - Top with the other bread slice, mustard side down.

- Cut the sandwich in half and enjoy!

## 4.  Vegetable and bean chili with tortilla chips and salsa:

- Ingredients:

  - 1 tablespoon of extra virgin olive oil

  - 1 onion, chopped

  - 2 carrots, peeled and diced

  - 2 celery stalks, sliced

  - 2 garlic cloves, minced

  - 1 teaspoon of dried thyme

  - 1 teaspoon of dried rosemary

  - 4 cups of vegetable broth

  - 2 cups of water

- 1 cup of brown or green lentils, rinsed and drained

- 1 bay leaf

- Salt and pepper to taste

- 2 cups of baby spinach leaves

- 2 tablespoons of lemon juice

- Tortilla chips, for serving

- Salsa, for serving

- Directions:

- In a large pot over medium-high heat, heat the oil and sauté the onion, carrot, celery, garlic, thyme, and rosemary for about 15 minutes, stirring occasionally, until the vegetables are soft and golden.

- Add the broth, water, lentils, bay leaf, salt, and pepper and bring to a boil. Reduce the heat and simmer, covered, for about 30 minutes or until the lentils are tender.

- Stir in the spinach and lemon juice and cook for another 5 minutes until the spinach is wilted.

- Discard the bay leaf and ladle the chili into bowls. Serve with tortilla chips and salsa on the side.

## 5. Tomato and mozzarella salad with balsamic dressing, whole wheat crackers, and grapes:

- For the salad, you will need the following ingredients:

    - 4 ripe plum tomatoes, sliced

    - 2 balls of fresh mozzarella cheese, sliced

    - A handful of fresh basil leaves

    - Salt and pepper to taste

- For the dressing, you will need the following ingredients:

    - 1/4 cup of extra virgin olive oil

- 3 tablespoons of balsamic vinegar

- 1 teaspoon of dried oregano

- 1/2 teaspoon of garlic powder

- For the crackers and grapes, you will need the following ingredients:

- Whole wheat crackers of your choice

- Fresh seedless grapes of your choice

- To make the salad, follow these steps:

- Arrange the tomato and mozzarella slices on a large platter, alternating them in a circular pattern. Sprinkle some salt and pepper over them.

- Tuck some basil leaves between the tomato and mozzarella slices. You can also tear some basil leaves and scatter them over the salad.

- To make the dressing, follow these steps:

    - In a small jar with a tight-fitting lid, shake the olive oil, balsamic vinegar, oregano, garlic powder, salt, and pepper until well combined.

    - Drizzle the dressing over the salad or serve it on the side.

- To serve the crackers and grapes, follow these steps:

    - Place some whole wheat crackers in a small bowl or plate.

    - Wash and dry some grapes and place them in another small bowl or plate.

- Enjoy your tomato and mozzarella salad with balsamic dressing, whole wheat crackers, and grapes!

**6.  Vegetable and cheese pizza on whole wheat crust:**

- For the crust, you will need the following ingredients:

- 1 1/4 cups of warm water

- 2 teaspoons of active dry yeast

- 1 teaspoon of honey

- 3 cups of whole wheat flour

- 1/4 cup of cornmeal

- 2 tablespoons of olive oil

- 1 teaspoon of salt

- For the toppings, you will need the following ingredients:

- 1 cup of pizza sauce or marinara sauce

- 2 cups of shredded mozzarella cheese

- 1/4 cup of grated Parmesan cheese

- 2 cups of assorted vegetables, such as mushrooms, bell

peppers, zucchini, broccoli, or spinach

- Optional: fresh basil leaves, red pepper flakes, or oregano for

garnish

- To make the pizza, follow these steps:

- In a large bowl, stir together the water, yeast, and honey. Let it sit for about 10 minutes or until foamy.

- Add the flour, cornmeal, oil, and salt and mix well. Turn the dough out onto a lightly floured surface and knead for about 15 minutes or until smooth and elastic. You can also use a stand mixer with a dough hook attachment to do this step.

- Place the dough in a lightly greased bowl and cover with a damp cloth. Let it rise in a warm place for about an hour or until doubled in size.

- Preheat the oven to 375°F and lightly grease a baking sheet or pizza pan.

- Punch down the dough and roll it out into a large circle or rectangle, depending on the shape of your pan. Transfer the dough to the prepared pan and press it evenly with your fingers.

- Spread the sauce evenly over the dough, leaving a small border around the edges. Sprinkle the mozzarella and Parmesan cheeses over the sauce. Top with your desired vegetables.

- Bake for 20 to 25 minutes or until the cheese is melted and bubbly and the crust is golden brown.

- Cut into slices and serve hot with fresh basil, red pepper flakes, or oregano if desired.

**7. Chicken and vegetable soup with whole wheat roll:**

- For the soup, you will need the following ingredients:

  - 1 tablespoon of extra virgin olive oil

  - 1 onion, chopped

  - 2 carrots, peeled and diced

  - 2 celery stalks, sliced

- 2 garlic cloves, minced

- 4 cups of chicken broth

- 2 cups of water

- 1 bay leaf

- Salt and pepper to taste

- 2 cups of cooked chicken, shredded or chopped

- 2 cups of mixed vegetables, such as green beans, corn, peas, or zucchini

- Fresh parsley, chopped, for garnish

- For the whole wheat roll, you will need the following ingredients:

- 1/4 cup of warm water

- 2 teaspoons of active dry yeast

- 1 teaspoon of honey

- 3 cups of whole wheat flour

- 1 teaspoon of salt

- 1/4 cup of melted butter

- 1 cup of milk

- To make the soup, follow these steps:

- In a large pot over medium-high heat, heat the oil and sauté the onion, carrot, celery, and garlic for about 15 minutes, stirring occasionally, until the vegetables are soft and golden.

- Add the broth, water, bay leaf, salt, and pepper and bring to a boil. Reduce the heat and simmer, covered, for about 20 minutes or until the carrots are tender.

- Stir in the chicken and mixed vegetables and cook for another 10 minutes or until heated through.

- Sprinkle some parsley over each serving and enjoy!

- To make the whole wheat roll, follow these steps:

- In a small bowl, stir together the water, yeast, and honey. Let it sit for about 10 minutes or until foamy.

- In a large bowl, whisk together the flour and salt. Make a well in the center and pour in the melted butter and milk. Stir with a wooden spoon until a shaggy dough forms.

- Turn the dough out onto a lightly floured surface and knead for about 15 minutes or until smooth and elastic. You can also use a stand mixer with a dough hook attachment to do this step.

- Place the dough in a lightly greased bowl and cover with a damp cloth. Let it rise in a warm place for about an hour or until doubled in size.

- Preheat the oven to 375°F and lightly grease a baking sheet.

- Punch down the dough and divide it into 12 equal pieces. Shape each piece into a ball and place them on the prepared baking sheet. Cover them with a damp cloth and let them rise for another 30 minutes or until puffy.

- Bake for 15 to 20 minutes or until golden brown.

- Enjoy your whole wheat roll with some butter or jam if desired.

8.  **Tuna salad sandwich on whole wheat bread with lettuce, tomato, and mayo:**

- Ingredients:

  - 1 can (6 ounces) of tuna in water, drained

  - 1/4 cup of chopped celery

  - 2 tablespoons of mayonnaise

  - Salt and pepper to taste

  - 4 slices of whole wheat bread, toasted

  - 4 lettuce leaves

  - 2 tomato slices

- Directions:

- In a small bowl, flake the tuna with a fork and mix it with the celery, mayonnaise, salt, and pepper.

- Spread the tuna mixture evenly over two slices of bread.

- Top each slice with two lettuce leaves and one tomato slice.

- Cover with the remaining bread slices and cut in half.

- Enjoy your tuna salad sandwich!

## 9. Vegetable lasagna with ricotta cheese, tomato sauce, and spinach:

- Ingredients:

- 9 lasagna noodles, cooked according to package directions

- 2 tablespoons of olive oil

- 1 onion, chopped

- 2 garlic cloves, minced

- 4 cups of fresh spinach, washed and chopped

- 2 cups of ricotta cheese

- 1/4 cup of grated Parmesan cheese

- 1 egg, lightly beaten

- Salt and pepper to taste

- 4 cups of tomato sauce (you can make your own or use a store-bought one)

- 2 cups of shredded mozzarella cheese

- Directions:

- Preheat the oven to 375°F and lightly grease a 9x13 inch baking dish.

- In a large skillet over medium-high heat, heat the oil and sauté the onion and garlic for about 15 minutes, stirring occasionally, until soft and golden.

- Add the spinach and cook for another 5 minutes, until wilted. Drain any excess liquid and set aside.

- In a medium bowl, stir together the ricotta cheese, Parmesan cheese, egg, salt, and pepper.

- To assemble the lasagna, spread about 1 cup of tomato sauce over the bottom of the prepared baking dish. Arrange 3 noodles over the sauce. Spread half of the ricotta mixture over the noodles. Sprinkle half of the spinach mixture over the ricotta. Repeat with another layer of sauce, noodles, ricotta, and spinach. Top with the remaining sauce and noodles. Sprinkle the mozzarella cheese evenly over the top.

- Bake for 25 to 30 minutes or until the cheese is melted and bubbly.

- Let the lasagna rest for 10 minutes before cutting and serving.

**10. Quinoa salad with chickpeas, tomatoes, cucumbers, parsley, lemon juice, and olive oil:**

- Ingredients:

    - 1 cup of uncooked quinoa, rinsed and drained

    - 2 cups of water

    - 1/4 teaspoon of salt

    - 1 can (15 ounces) of chickpeas, rinsed and drained, or 1 1/2
cups cooked chickpeas

    - 2 cups of cherry tomatoes, halved

    - 1 large cucumber, peeled and diced

    - 1/4 cup of sliced black olives

    - 1/4 cup of chopped fresh parsley

    - 3 tablespoons of lemon juice

    - 3 tablespoons of extra virgin olive oil

- Salt and pepper to taste

- Directions:

- In a medium saucepan, bring the quinoa, water, and salt to a boil. Reduce the heat and simmer, covered, until the quinoa is fluffy and the water is absorbed, about 15 to 20 minutes. Fluff with a fork and let it cool slightly.

- In a large salad bowl, toss the chickpeas, tomatoes, cucumber, olives, and parsley together.

- In a small jar with a tight-fitting lid, shake the lemon juice, olive oil, salt, and pepper until well combined.

- Add the quinoa and dressing to the salad and toss to coat. Adjust the seasoning if needed.

- Enjoy your quinoa salad as a main or a side dish. You can also refrigerate it for up to 4 days.

**11. Minestrone soup with parmesan cheese and whole wheat breadstick:**

Ingredients:

- 4 tablespoons extra-virgin olive oil, divided

- 1 medium yellow onion, chopped

- 2 medium carrots, peeled and chopped

- 2 medium ribs celery, chopped

- ¼ cup tomato paste

- 2 cups chopped seasonal vegetables (potatoes, yellow squash, zucchini, butternut squash, green beans or peas all work)

- 4 cloves garlic, pressed or minced

- ½ teaspoon dried oregano

- ½ teaspoon dried thyme

- 1 large can (28 ounces) diced tomatoes, with their liquid (or 2 small 15-ounce cans)

- 4 cups (32 ounces) vegetable broth

- 2 cups water

- 1 teaspoon fine sea salt

- 2 bay leaves

- Pinch of red pepper flakes

- Freshly ground black pepper

- 1 cup whole grain orecchiette, elbow or small shell pasta

- 1 can (15 ounces) kidney beans, rinsed and drained, or 1 ½ cups cooked kidney beans

- 2 cups baby spinach or chopped kale

- 2 teaspoons lemon juice

- Freshly grated Parmesan cheese, for garnishing

Instructions:

1. In a large pot over medium-high heat, warm 3 tablespoons of the olive oil until shimmering. Add the onion, carrot, celery and a pinch of salt. Cook, stirring occasionally, until the vegetables are tender, about 15 minutes.

2. Stir in the tomato paste, garlic, oregano and thyme and cook for another minute, stirring constantly.

3. Add the diced tomatoes and their juices, broth, water, salt, bay leaves and red pepper flakes. Raise the heat and bring the mixture to a boil, then partially cover the pot with the lid, leaving some room for steam to escape. Reduce the heat as necessary to maintain a gentle simmer.

4. Add the pasta and cook until al dente, about 10 to 15 minutes, stirring occasionally. Add the beans and spinach and stir until the spinach wilts, about 2 minutes. Remove the pot from the heat and discard the bay leaves.

5. Stir in the lemon juice and remaining 1 tablespoon of olive oil.

Taste and season with more salt and pepper as needed.

6. Ladle the soup into bowls and top with grated Parmesan cheese.

Enjoy!


For the whole wheat breadstick, you can follow this simple recipe

or use store-bought ones if you prefer.


12. **Roasted vegetable sandwich on whole wheat bread with
    hummus,**


Ingredients:

- 2 slices of whole wheat bread

- 1/4 cup of hummus (preferably jalapeno-cilantro flavor)

- 2 tablespoons of crumbled feta cheese

- 1/4 cup of sliced peppadew peppers (see Tip)

- 1/4 cup of sliced cucumber

- 2 slices of tomato

- 2 thin slices of red onion

- A handful of lettuce leaves (any kind you like)

- Salt and pepper to taste

Directions:

1. Preheat the oven to 350°F and line a baking sheet with

parchment paper. Arrange the sliced peppers, cucumber, tomato

and onion on the prepared sheet and drizzle with some olive oil.

Sprinkle with salt and pepper and roast for about 25 minutes, or until the vegetables are tender and slightly charred.

2. Toast the bread lightly, if desired, and spread hummus evenly on both slices. Sprinkle feta cheese on one slice and top with the roasted vegetables. Add the lettuce leaves and close the sandwich with the other slice of bread.

3. Cut the sandwich in half and enjoy!

Tip: Peppadew peppers are small, sweet and spicy peppers that add a burst of flavor to this sandwich. You can find them at the olive bar in most grocery stores or online[1].

I hope you like this recipe!

**13. Nicoise salad with tuna, hard-boiled eggs, potatoes, green beans, olives, and vinaigrette dressing**

Ingredients:

- 4 medium Yukon Gold potatoes, peeled and cut into 1-inch pieces

- Salt and black pepper

- 4 large eggs

- 8 ounces green beans, trimmed and halved

- 1/4 cup extra virgin olive oil

- 3 tablespoons red wine vinegar

- 2 teaspoons Dijon mustard

- 1 garlic clove, minced

- 2 (5-ounce) cans tuna in water, drained and flaked

- 8 cups mixed salad greens

- 2 medium tomatoes, cut into wedges

- 1/4 cup pitted black olives (preferably Niçoise or Kalamata)

- Optional: 2 tablespoons capers and/or 8 anchovy fillets

Directions:

1. In a large pot of boiling salted water, cook the potatoes until tender, about 15 to 20 minutes. Drain and transfer to a large bowl. Sprinkle with salt and pepper to taste.

2. In a small saucepan of boiling water, cook the eggs until hard-boiled, about 10 minutes. Drain and run under cold water to stop the cooking. Peel and quarter the eggs.

3. In a medium pot of boiling salted water, cook the green beans until crisp-tender, about 5 minutes. Drain and rinse under cold water to cool.

4. In a small bowl, whisk together the olive oil, vinegar, mustard, garlic, salt and pepper to make the vinaigrette dressing.

5. To assemble the salad, arrange the greens on a large platter. Top with the potatoes, eggs, green beans, tuna, tomatoes and olives. Drizzle with some of the dressing and toss lightly to coat. Sprinkle with capers and/or anchovies if using. Serve with more dressing on the side or refrigerate until ready to serve.

## SNACKS

1. **Hummus with carrot and celery sticks is a simple and healthy snack that you can make at home.**

Ingredients:

- 1/4 cup hummus (preferably jalapeno-cilantro flavor)

- 1 carrot, cut into dipping sticks

- 2 celery stalks, cut into dipping sticks

Directions:

1. Dip the carrot and celery sticks in the hummus and enjoy!

**2.  Greek yogurt with honey and walnuts**

 is a traditional Greek dessert that is simple, healthy and delicious. It is made by combining thick and creamy Greek yogurt with sweet honey and crunchy walnuts. You can also add some fresh fruit or granola for extra flavor and texture.

Ingredients:

- 4 cups of Greek yogurt (preferably full-fat and plain or vanilla flavored)

- 1/2 cup of walnuts (toasted and chopped)

- 3 tablespoons of honey (preferably organic and thyme flavored)

- Optional: fresh fruit (such as berries, peaches, figs or pomegranate seeds) or low-fat granola

Directions:

1. In a large bowl, whisk the yogurt until smooth and creamy.

2. In a small bowl, toss the walnuts with 1 tablespoon of honey.

3. Divide the yogurt among four serving bowls or glasses.

4. Drizzle the remaining honey over the yogurt.

5. Sprinkle the walnut mixture on top.

6. Add some fresh fruit or granola if desired.

7. Enjoy!

## 3.  Orange Almond Cake:

Ingredients:

- 1 large orange

- 1 cup white sugar

- 3 eggs

- 1 teaspoon baking powder

- 2 cups almond flour

- 1/4 cup butter, melted

- Powdered sugar for dusting

Directions:

1. Preheat oven to 375 degrees F (190 degrees C). Grease a 9-inch springform pan.

2. Cut the orange into quarters and remove any seeds. Place the orange pieces in a large pot of water and bring to a boil. Cook until very soft, about 30 minutes. Drain and let cool slightly.

3. Transfer the orange pieces to a food processor and puree with the sugar until smooth. Add the eggs and pulse to combine. Add the baking powder and almond flour and pulse until well blended. Add the butter and pulse until incorporated.

4. Pour the batter into the prepared pan and smooth the top. Bake for 35 to 45 minutes or until a toothpick inserted in the center comes out clean.

5. Let the cake cool completely in the pan on a wire rack. Run a knife around the edge of the pan and remove the side. Dust with powdered sugar before serving.

## 4. **Roasted chickpeas**

Ingredients:

- 1 (15 ounce) can chickpeas (garbanzo beans), drained

- 2 tablespoons olive oil

- 1 pinch garlic salt, or to taste

- 1 pinch cayenne pepper, or to taste

- 1 pinch salt, or to taste

Directions:

1. Preheat oven to 375 degrees F (190 degrees C). Grease a 9-inch springform pan.

2. Cut the orange into quarters and remove any seeds. Place the orange pieces in a large pot of water and bring to a boil. Cook until very soft, about 30 minutes. Drain and let cool slightly.

3. Transfer the orange pieces to a food processor and puree with the sugar until smooth. Add the eggs and pulse to combine. Add the baking powder and almond flour and pulse until well blended. Add the butter and pulse until incorporated.

4. Pour the batter into the prepared pan and smooth the top. Bake for 35 to 45 minutes or until a toothpick inserted in the center comes out clean.

5. Let the cake cool completely in the pan on a wire rack. Run a knife around the edge of the pan and remove the side. Dust with powdered sugar before serving.

## 5.  Greek yogurt dip with fresh veggies

Ingredients:

- 2 cups plain Greek yogurt

- 1/4 cup chopped fresh dill

- 2 tablespoons lemon juice

- 2 cloves garlic, minced

- Salt and pepper to taste

Directions:

1. In a small bowl, whisk together the yogurt, dill, lemon juice, garlic, salt and pepper until well combined.

2. Refrigerate the dip for at least 30 minutes to let the flavors meld.

3. Serve with your favorite fresh vegetables, such as carrots, celery, cucumber, bell pepper, cherry tomatoes or broccoli.

6. **Mediterranean pinwheels**

Ingredients:

- 6 large tortillas (spinach or sun-dried tomato flavor recommended)

- 8 ounces cream cheese

- A pinch of salt and black pepper

- 2 tablespoons pre-minced garlic (or fresh)

- 6 ounces sun-dried tomatoes (in oil, chopped and oil reserved)

- 12 ounces spinach (frozen, cooked, water squeezed out, chopped)

- 1/4 cup Parmesan cheese (grated)

- 1/3 cup feta cheese (crumbles)

- 1 cup fresh basil leaves


Directions:


1. In a small bowl, mix the cream cheese with salt, pepper and garlic until smooth. Add some oil from the sun-dried tomatoes if needed to thin it out.

2. Spread a thin layer of the cream cheese mixture over each tortilla, leaving a 1/2 inch border around the edges.

3. Sprinkle the sun-dried tomatoes, spinach, Parmesan cheese and feta cheese evenly over the cream cheese layer.

4. Top with basil leaves and roll up the tortillas tightly.

5. Wrap each tortilla roll in plastic wrap and refrigerate for at least an hour or up to overnight.

6. Cut into 1-inch slices and serve.

**7. Dried figs and pistachios**

Ingredients:

- 1 cup all-purpose flour

- 1 cup whole wheat flour

- 1/2 cup brown sugar

- 2 teaspoons baking soda

- 1/2 teaspoon salt

- 1/2 cup raisins

- 1/2 cup shelled pistachios

- 1/4 cup sesame seeds

- 1/4 cup flax seeds

- 1/4 cup sunflower seeds

- 2 cups plain Greek yogurt

- 1/4 cup honey

- 1/4 cup molasses

- 1 cup chopped dried figs

Directions:

1. Preheat oven to 350°F and spray two loaf pans with cooking

spray.

2. Combine both flours, brown sugar, baking soda and salt in a large mixing bowl. Add raisins, pistachios and all seeds. Stir to mix well.

3. In a small bowl, whisk together yogurt, honey and molasses. Add to the dry ingredients and stir until all flour is incorporated. Add chopped figs and stir gently just to combine.

4. Divide the batter evenly between the two prepared pans and smooth the tops. Bake for 25 to 30 minutes or until a toothpick inserted in the center comes out clean.

5. Let the loaves cool completely in the pans on a wire rack. Wrap them tightly in plastic wrap and refrigerate for at least two hours or up to two days.

6. Preheat oven to 300°F and line two baking sheets with parchment paper. Cut each loaf into thin slices, about 1/8 inch thick, using a serrated knife. Place the slices on the prepared baking sheets in a single layer.

7. Bake for 15 minutes, then flip the slices over and bake for another 10 minutes or until crisp and golden. Let them cool completely on the baking sheets.

8. Enjoy your fig and pistachio crisps as they are or with cheese, jam or honey.

**8.  Celery sticks with cream cheese**

Ingredients:

- 1 bunch of celery, washed and trimmed

- 1/4 cup of cream cheese, softened

- 2 tablespoons of raisins

Directions:

1. Cut the celery stalks into 3-inch pieces and pat them dry with paper towels.

2. In a small bowl, stir the cream cheese until smooth and creamy.

3. Spoon the cream cheese into a piping bag or a ziplock bag with one corner snipped off.

4. Pipe the cream cheese into the hollow part of each celery piece, filling it generously.

5. Sprinkle the raisins over the cream cheese filling, pressing them lightly to stick.

6. Enjoy your celery sticks with cream cheese and raisins as a snack or appetizer.

**DINNER**

**1. Baked salmon with lemon and herbs, roasted asparagus, and brown rice:**

Ingredients:

- 4 (6-ounce) salmon fillets

- Salt and pepper to taste

- 2 tablespoons of olive oil

- 2 tablespoons of lemon juice

- 2 teaspoons of minced garlic

- 1 teaspoon of dried oregano

- 1/4 teaspoon of paprika

- 2 tablespoons of chopped fresh parsley

- 1 pound of asparagus, trimmed

- 4 lemon slices

- 2 cups of brown rice

- 4 cups of water or broth

- Optional: butter, cheese, or your favorite sauce for serving


Directions:


1. Preheat oven to 375°F and line a baking sheet with foil. Spray with cooking spray or brush with some oil.

2. Season the salmon fillets with salt and pepper on both sides and place them on the prepared baking sheet, skin-side down.

3. In a small bowl, whisk together the olive oil, lemon juice, garlic, oregano, paprika, and parsley. Spoon the mixture over the salmon fillets, making sure to coat them well.

4. Arrange the asparagus around the salmon on the same baking sheet. Drizzle with some more oil and season with salt and pepper. Place a lemon slice on top of each salmon fillet.

5. Bake for 15 to 20 minutes or until the salmon is cooked through and flakes easily with a fork. The asparagus should be tender but crisp.

6. While the salmon and asparagus are baking, cook the brown rice according to the package directions. You can use water or broth for more flavor. Fluff with a fork when done and keep warm until ready to serve.

7. Serve the baked salmon and asparagus with the brown rice on the side. You can also add some butter, cheese, or your favorite sauce if you like.

**2.  Vegetable and cheese frittata with whole wheat**

Ingredients:

- 8 eggs

- 1/4 cup milk

- Salt and pepper to taste

- 2 tablespoons butter

- 1 onion, chopped

- 2 cups chopped spinach

- 1/4 cup chopped fresh basil

- 1 cup shredded mozzarella cheese

- 4 slices of whole wheat bread

Directions:

1. Preheat oven to 375°F and lightly grease a 9-inch pie dish.

2. In a medium bowl, whisk together the eggs, milk, salt and

pepper until well combined. Set aside.

3. In a large skillet over medium-high heat, melt the butter and cook the onion until soft, about 10 minutes. Add the spinach and basil and cook until wilted, stirring occasionally, about 5 minutes.

4. Transfer the onion and spinach mixture to the prepared pie dish and spread it evenly. Sprinkle the cheese on top.

5. Pour the egg mixture over the cheese and vegetable layer, making sure to cover them well.

6. Bake for 25 to 30 minutes or until the eggs are set and golden on the edges.

7. Toast the bread slices in a toaster or oven until crisp and lightly browned.

8. Cut the frittata into wedges and serve with the toast.

**3. Spaghetti with tomato and basil sauce, green salad, and garlic bread**

Here is a possible recipe for spaghetti with tomato and basil sauce, green salad, and garlic bread that I created based on the web search results:

Ingredients:

- 1 pound of spaghetti

- 4 tablespoons of olive oil, divided

- 4 cloves of garlic, minced, divided

- 1/4 teaspoon of red pepper flakes (optional)

- 4 cups of cherry tomatoes, halved

- Salt and pepper to taste

- 1/4 cup of fresh basil leaves, chopped

- 1/4 cup of grated Parmesan cheese

- 4 slices of whole wheat bread

- 2 tablespoons of butter, softened

- 1 teaspoon of dried parsley

- 1/4 teaspoon of garlic powder

- 4 cups of mixed salad greens

- 1/4 cup of your favorite salad dressing

Directions:

1. Cook the spaghetti in a large pot of boiling salted water according to the package directions, until al dente. Drain and return to the pot. Keep warm.

2. In a large skillet over medium-high heat, heat 2 tablespoons of olive oil and cook 2 cloves of garlic and red pepper flakes (if using) for about a minute, stirring frequently. Add the cherry tomatoes and season with salt and pepper. Cook for about 15 minutes, stirring occasionally, until the tomatoes are soft and juicy. Stir in the basil and remove from the heat.

3. Preheat the oven to 375°F and line a baking sheet with foil. In a small bowl, combine the butter, parsley, garlic powder, and a pinch of salt. Spread the butter mixture evenly over the bread slices and place them on the prepared baking sheet. Bake for about 10 minutes or until golden and crisp.

4. In a large bowl, toss the salad greens with the remaining 2 tablespoons of olive oil and your favorite salad dressing. Season with salt and pepper if needed.

5. Serve the spaghetti topped with the tomato and basil sauce and sprinkled with Parmesan cheese. Serve with the garlic bread and the green salad on the side.

## **4. Shrimp and vegetable stir-fry with brown rice**

Ingredients:

- 2 cups instant brown rice

- 1 ¾ cups water

- 6 tablespoons soy sauce

- 6 tablespoons water

- ¼ cup honey

- 2 tablespoons cider vinegar

- 2 tablespoons cornstarch

- 2 tablespoons olive oil

- 2 cloves garlic, chopped

- 2 cups broccoli florets

- 1 cup baby carrots

- 1 small white onion, chopped

- ½ teaspoon black pepper

- 1 cup sliced fresh mushrooms

- 1 ½ pounds uncooked medium shrimp, peeled and deveined

Directions:

1. Stir rice and water together in a microwave-safe bowl. Cover and cook in the microwave on high until water is fully absorbed, about 8 minutes. Fluff with a fork; cover and set aside.

2. Whisk together soy sauce, water, honey, cider vinegar, and cornstarch in a small bowl; set sauce mixture aside.

3. Heat olive oil in a nonstick skillet or wok over medium heat. Stir in garlic and cook for 10 seconds. Add broccoli, carrots, onion, and black pepper; cook and stir until broccoli and carrots are tender, about 5 minutes.

4. Stir in mushrooms and cook for 2 minutes. Remove vegetables from the skillet and set aside.

5. Return the skillet to heat and pour in sauce mixture; cook for 1 minute. Add shrimp and stir until shrimp are bright pink on the outside, meat is no longer transparent, and sauce thickens, about 3 minutes.

6. Stir vegetables into the pan and serve over brown rice.

**5. Lamb chops with mint sauce, couscous, and roasted carrots**

Ingredients:

- 4 lamb chops or leg steaks, trimmed

- Salt and pepper, to taste

- 2 tbsp olive oil

- 4 cloves garlic, minced

- 1/4 cup rice vinegar

- 2 tbsp soy sauce

- 1 tsp sesame oil

- 1/4 tsp red chili flakes

- 1/4 cup fresh mint, chopped

- 200 g couscous

- 5 tbsp pine nuts, toasted

- 8 dates, pitted and chopped

- Zest and juice of 2 lemons

- 20 g fresh parsley, chopped

- Cooking spray or oil, for greasing

- 4 large carrots, peeled and cut into thin slices

- 2 tbsp honey

- 2 tbsp butter, melted


Directions:


1. To make the mint sauce, whisk together the garlic, rice vinegar, soy sauce, sesame oil, red chili flakes, and mint in a small bowl. Set aside.

2. To make the couscous, boil some water in a kettle and place the couscous in a heatproof bowl. Stir in the pine nuts, dates, lemon zest, and half of the lemon juice. Pour over enough boiling water to just cover the couscous. Cover the bowl with a plate and let it

stand for 10 minutes. Fluff with a fork and stir in half of the parsley. Season with salt and pepper to taste.

3. To make the roasted carrots, preheat the oven to 200°C (180°C fan) and line a baking sheet with parchment paper. Toss the carrot slices with the honey and butter in a large bowl. Spread them in an even layer on the prepared baking sheet. Bake for 25 to 30 minutes or until tender and caramelized.

4. To cook the lamb chops, heat a grill pan over high heat until almost smoking. Season the lamb chops with salt and pepper on both sides. Spray the grill pan with some cooking spray or brush with some oil. Add the lamb chops and cook for 2 to 3 minutes per side or until done to your liking. Transfer to a platter and let them rest for 10 minutes, covered with foil.

5. To serve, divide the couscous among four plates and top with a lamb chop each. Drizzle some of the mint sauce over the lamb and couscous. Serve with the roasted carrots on the side. Sprinkle some more parsley over everything if desired. Enjoy!

## 6.  Ratatouille (vegetable stew) with crusty bread

Ingredients:

- 1/4 cup extra virgin olive oil, plus more for drizzling

- 1 large onion, diced

- 4 cloves garlic, minced

- 1 large eggplant, cut into 2 cm / 4/5" cubes

- 2 zucchinis, cut into 2 cm / 4/5" cubes

- 2 red or yellow bell peppers, cut into 2 cm / 4/5" pieces

- 800 g / 28 oz canned crushed tomatoes

- 2 tsp dried thyme or 3 sprigs fresh thyme

- Salt and pepper, to taste

- 1/4 cup fresh basil leaves, chopped, plus more for garnish

Directions:

1. Heat oil in a large pot over medium-high heat. Add onion and garlic and cook, stirring occasionally, for about 15 minutes or until onion is soft and golden.

2. Add eggplant and cook, stirring occasionally, for another 15 minutes or until eggplant is soft and browned.

3. Add zucchini and bell peppers and cook, stirring occasionally, for another 10 minutes or until slightly softened.

4. Add tomatoes, thyme, salt and pepper and bring to a boil. Reduce heat and simmer, uncovered, for about 20 minutes or until vegetables are tender and sauce is slightly thickened.

5. Stir through basil then serve immediately, drizzled with extra

virgin olive oil and a sprinkle of extra basil on top, if desired.

Serve with crusty bread to mop up the sauce. Enjoy! ☐

## 7.  Roasted pork loin with apple sauce, mashed potatoes, and broccoli

Ingredients:

- 1 boneless pork loin roast (3 pounds), trimmed and tied

- Salt and pepper, to taste

- 2 tablespoons vegetable oil

- 1/4 cup applesauce

- 3 tablespoons Dijon mustard

- 1 tablespoon honey

- 3 fresh rosemary sprigs

- 1 cup chicken broth, low-sodium or homemade

- 1 to 2 tablespoons whole grain mustard

- 1 to 2 tablespoons unsalted butter, diced and chilled

- 4 large potatoes, peeled and cut into chunks

- 1/4 cup milk, warmed

- 2 tablespoons sour cream

- 4 cups broccoli florets

- 2 tablespoons water

Directions:

1. Preheat the oven to 350°F. Sprinkle the pork loin with salt and

pepper on all sides. In a large ovenproof skillet, heat the oil over medium-high heat. Brown the pork on all sides, about 2 to 3 minutes per side. Transfer the pork to a plate and set aside.

2. In a small bowl, whisk together the applesauce, Dijon mustard, and honey. Spread the mixture over the pork and top with rosemary sprigs. Return the pork to the skillet and add the chicken broth. Transfer the skillet to the oven and roast for about 40 minutes or until a thermometer inserted into the center of the meat reads between 145°F to 150°F. Transfer the pork to a cutting board and tent with foil. Let it rest for 10 minutes before slicing.

3. Meanwhile, place the potatoes in a large pot of salted water and bring to a boil. Cook until tender, about 15 to 20 minutes. Drain and return to the pot. Mash the potatoes with a potato masher or an electric mixer. Add the milk, sour cream, butter, salt and pepper and mix well.

4. In a microwave-safe bowl, combine the broccoli and water. Cover with plastic wrap and microwave on high for about 5

minutes or until crisp-tender. Drain and season with salt and pepper.

5. To make the sauce, strain the cooking liquid from the skillet into a small saucepan. Bring to a boil over high heat and reduce by about a third. Whisk in the whole grain mustard and butter. Season with salt and pepper to taste.

6. To serve, divide the mashed potatoes among four plates and top with sliced pork. Drizzle some sauce over the meat and potatoes. Serve with broccoli on the side. Enjoy! □

8. **Fish tacos with cabbage slaw, avocado, salsa, and sour cream:**

Ingredients:

- 1 pound white fish fillets, such as tilapia, cod, or halibut

- 1/4 teaspoon salt

- 1/4 teaspoon black pepper

- 2 tablespoons canola oil

- 8 corn tortillas, warmed

- 1 ripe avocado, peeled and sliced

- 1/4 cup salsa of your choice

- 1/4 cup sour cream

For the slaw:

- 2 cups shredded red or green cabbage

- 1/4 cup chopped fresh cilantro

- 2 tablespoons lime juice

- 1 tablespoon honey

- 1/4 teaspoon cumin

- 1/4 teaspoon salt

- 1/4 teaspoon black pepper

- 1/4 teaspoon red pepper flakes (optional)

Directions:

1. To make the slaw, toss the cabbage and cilantro in a large bowl. In a small bowl, whisk together the lime juice, honey, cumin, salt, black pepper, and red pepper flakes if using. Drizzle over the cabbage mixture and toss to coat. Refrigerate until ready to serve.

2. To cook the fish, season the fillets with salt and pepper on both sides. Heat the oil in a large nonstick skillet over medium-high heat. Cook the fish for about 3 to 4 minutes per side or until golden and flaky. Transfer to a plate and break into bite-sized pieces.

3. To assemble the tacos, divide the fish among the tortillas and top with the slaw, avocado slices, salsa, and sour cream. Enjoy! □

## 9.  Mushroom risotto with parmesan cheese, green salad

Ingredients:

- 6 cups chicken broth, divided

- 3 tablespoons olive oil, divided

- 1 pound portobello mushrooms, thinly sliced

- 1 pound white mushrooms, thinly sliced

- 2 shallots, diced

- 1 1/2 cups Arborio rice

- 1/2 cup dry white wine

- Sea salt and black pepper, to taste

- 3 tablespoons finely chopped chives

- 4 tablespoons butter

- 1/3 cup freshly grated Parmesan cheese

For the green salad:

- 4 cups mixed greens, washed and dried

- 1/4 cup cherry tomatoes, halved

- 2 tablespoons sliced almonds, toasted

- 2 tablespoons balsamic vinegar

- 2 tablespoons olive oil

- Salt and pepper, to taste

Directions:

1. In a saucepan, warm the chicken broth over low heat.

2. In a large skillet over medium-high heat, heat 2 tablespoons of olive oil. Add the mushrooms and cook, stirring occasionally, until tender and browned, about 15 minutes. Transfer the mushrooms and their liquid to a bowl and set aside.

3. In the same skillet over medium heat, heat the remaining tablespoon of olive oil. Add the shallots and cook, stirring occasionally, until soft, about 5 minutes. Add the rice and cook, stirring constantly, until well coated with oil, about 2 minutes. Add the wine and simmer until almost evaporated, scraping up any browned bits from the bottom of the pan, about 3 minutes.

4. Add 1/2 cup of the warm broth and stir until almost completely absorbed, about 2 minutes. Continue adding the broth, 1/2 cup at a time, stirring constantly and allowing each addition to absorb

before adding the next, until the rice is al dente and creamy, about 20 minutes. Season with salt and pepper to taste.

5. Stir in the mushrooms with their liquid, chives, butter, and Parmesan cheese. Adjust the seasoning if needed.

6. To make the green salad, toss the greens, tomatoes, and almonds in a large bowl. In a small bowl, whisk together the vinegar, oil, salt and pepper. Drizzle over the salad and toss to coat.

7. To serve, divide the risotto among four plates and top with more Parmesan cheese if desired. Serve with the green salad on the side. Enjoy! □

**10.Moroccan tagine (stew) with lamb, chickpeas, apricots, and almonds, couscous**

Ingredients:

- 1 kg lamb neck fillet, cut into large chunks

- 3 tbsp ras el hanout

- Salt and pepper, to taste

- 2 tbsp olive oil

- 2 onions, chopped

- 4 carrots, cut into large chunks

- 6 garlic cloves, finely chopped

- Thumb-sized piece of ginger, peeled and finely grated

- 2 tbsp rose harissa paste, plus 1 tsp to serve

- 1/2 preserved lemon, finely chopped, or a peeled strip of lemon

zest

- 1 cinnamon stick

- 400 g can chopped tomatoes

- 600 ml chicken or lamb stock

- 2 x 400 g cans chickpeas, drained but not rinsed

- 100 g dried apricots, roughly chopped (optional)

- 150 g natural yogurt

- Small bunch of coriander, roughly chopped

- Small handful of flaked almonds, toasted

- Cooked couscous

Directions:

1. Toss the lamb pieces with the ras el hanout and a large pinch of salt to coat. Will keep chilled for up to 4 hrs. Heat the oven to 160°C/140°C fan/gas 3. Heat the oil in a large flameproof casserole over a medium heat and brown the lamb on all sides, about 4 minutes per batch. Transfer the lamb to a plate and set aside.

2. Add the onion and carrots to the same casserole and cook over a medium heat, stirring occasionally, for about 15 minutes or until soft and golden. Add the garlic and ginger and cook for another 2 minutes. Stir in the 2 tbsp harissa and preserved lemon. Cook for another minute until the vegetables are coated in the mixture and sticky. Add the cinnamon stick and tomatoes and bring to a simmer.

3. Cook for a few minutes more until reduced to a thick paste. Return the lamb and any juices back to the casserole and pour over the stock. Season with salt and pepper and bring to a simmer. Cover with a lid and transfer to the oven for 1 hour.

4. Stir in the chickpeas and apricots if using. Cover again and return to the oven for another hour until the lamb is tender.

5. Swirl the remaining tsp of harissa through the yogurt. Sprinkle the tagine with coriander and almonds. Serve with couscous and yogurt on the side. Enjoy!

## 11. Paella (rice dish) with shrimp, chicken, sausage, and peas:

Ingredients:

- 1 cup of Arborio rice or Spanish bomba rice

- 1/2 pound of raw shrimp, peeled and deveined

- 2 medium chicken sausages, chopped into bite-sized pieces

- 1/4 cup of frozen green peas

- 2 cups of seafood stock or chicken broth

- 1/2 white onion, diced

- 2 cloves of garlic, minced

- 1/4 cup of diccd tomato

- 3 tablespoons of olive oil

- 1 teaspoon of smoked paprika

- 1/4 teaspoon of red chili powder

- A pinch of saffron threads or turmeric

- Salt and pepper, to taste

- Fresh parsley, chopped, for garnish

To make the paella, follow these steps:

1. In a large ovenproof skillet over medium-high heat, heat 2 tablespoons of olive oil. Season the chicken sausage with salt, pepper, and half of the paprika and chili powder. Cook for about 10 minutes, turning occasionally, until browned. Transfer to a plate and set aside.

2. In the same skillet over medium-high heat, heat the remaining tablespoon of olive oil. Season the shrimp with salt, pepper, and the remaining paprika and chili powder. Cook for about 3 minutes per side, until pink and curled. Transfer to a plate and set aside.

3. Preheat the oven to 400°F. In the same skillet over medium heat, add the onion and garlic and cook, stirring occasionally, for about 15 minutes or until soft and golden. Add the rice and cook, stirring constantly, for about 2 minutes or until well coated with oil.

4. Stir in the tomato, saffron or turmeric, salt and pepper. Pour in the stock or broth and bring to a boil. Reduce the heat and simmer, uncovered, for about 15 minutes or until the rice is almost tender but still firm to the bite.

5. Arrange the chicken sausage and shrimp over the rice. Sprinkle the peas over the top. Cover the skillet with foil and bake for about 10 minutes or until the rice is fully cooked and the liquid is absorbed.

6. Sprinkle with parsley and serve hot with lemon wedges if desired.

**CHAPTER 5: TIPS AND TRICKS FOR STICKING TO THE MEDITERRANEAN DIET: how to eat out, travel, and deal with cravings**

The Mediterranean diet is a healthy eating pattern that is based on the traditional foods of countries that border the Mediterranean Sea. It is rich in plant foods, healthy fats, and moderate amounts of fish, poultry, dairy, and wine. It has been shown to have many benefits for your health, such as reducing the risk of heart disease, diabetes, and some cancers.

However, following the Mediterranean diet can be challenging for some people, especially when they are eating out, traveling, or dealing with cravings. Here are some tips and tricks to help you stick to the Mediterranean diet in different situations:

- When eating out, look for dishes that feature vegetables, whole grains, legumes, nuts, and olive oil. Avoid fried foods, creamy sauces, and processed meats. Choose fish or seafood over red meat, and limit cheese and butter. Ask for salad dressing on the side, and use olive oil and vinegar instead. For dessert, opt for fresh fruit or a small piece of dark chocolate.

- When traveling, pack some healthy snacks that are easy to carry and store, such as nuts, dried fruits, whole-grain crackers, or granola bars. You can also buy fresh fruits and vegetables from local markets or grocery stores. Try to avoid fast food and convenience foods that are high in salt, sugar, and fat. Instead, look for restaurants that serve local cuisine that is similar to the Mediterranean diet, such as Greek, Turkish, Moroccan, or Lebanese food.

- When dealing with cravings, remember that the Mediterranean diet is not a strict or restrictive diet. You can enjoy occasional treats in moderation, as long as you balance them with healthy foods. For example, you can have a glass of red wine with your dinner, or a slice of cake at a birthday party. However, you should not overindulge or binge on unhealthy foods. If you crave something sweet or salty, try to satisfy your craving with a healthier alternative, such as a piece of fruit, a handful of nuts, or some hummus with carrot sticks.

# CHAPTER 6: FAQS ON MEDITERRANEAN DIET

Some frequently asked questions about the Mediterranean diet and answers to common concerns and misconceptions are:

- What is the Mediterranean diet and where does it come from?

- The Mediterranean diet is a healthy eating pattern that is based on the traditional foods of countries that border the Mediterranean Sea, such as Italy, France, Greece, Croatia, and Spain. It is rich in plant foods, healthy fats, and moderate amounts of fish, poultry, dairy, and wine. It has been shown to have many benefits for your health, such as reducing the risk of heart disease, diabetes, and some cancers. The Mediterranean diet was not designed by a nutritionist or a dietician, but rather emerged naturally from the lifestyle and culture of the people living in the Mediterranean region.

- Is the Mediterranean diet good for weight loss?

- Yes, the Mediterranean diet can help you lose weight if you follow it along with regular physical activity. The Mediterranean diet is not a specific weight loss program, but rather a balanced and flavorful way of eating that can help you control your calorie intake and improve your metabolism. The diet is low in saturated fats and high in fruits, vegetables, whole grains, legumes, nuts, and olive oil, which can help you feel full and satisfied. However, you should still be mindful of your portion sizes and avoid overeating or bingeing on unhealthy foods.

- Do I need to watch my calories on the Mediterranean diet?

- No, the Mediterranean diet does not require you to count calories or measure your food. However, you should still be aware of how much you are eating and choose foods that are nutrient-dense and low in calories. For example, you should limit your intake of olive oil to no more than 3 tablespoons a day, as it is high in calories and fat. You should also avoid fried foods, creamy sauces, processed meats, added sugars, and refined grains[2]. Instead, you should focus on eating more vegetables, fruits, whole grains, legumes, nuts, seeds, fish, and seafood.

- Is the Mediterranean diet suitable for vegetarians or vegans?

- Yes, the Mediterranean diet can easily be adapted for vegetarians or vegans. The diet is already rich in plant-based foods that provide protein, fiber, vitamins, minerals, antioxidants, and phytochemicals. You can also include dairy products and eggs if you are a lacto-ovo vegetarian. If you are a vegan or want to avoid animal products altogether, you can get enough calcium and vitamin D from fortified soy beverages or other plant-based milks[3]. You can also supplement your diet with vitamin B12 if needed.

- Does the Mediterranean diet include a grocery list?

- No, the Mediterranean diet does not have a specific grocery list or shopping plan. However, you can use some general guidelines to help you stock your pantry and fridge with healthy foods that are typical of the Mediterranean diet. Some examples are:

- Vegetables: fresh or frozen vegetables of different colors and varieties, such as tomatoes, cucumbers, lettuce, spinach, kale, broccoli, cauliflower, carrots, peppers, eggplant, zucchini

- Fruits: fresh or dried fruits of different types and seasons

- Whole grains: whole wheat breads

- Legumes: beans

- Nuts: almonds

- Seeds: sunflower seeds

- Olive oil: extra virgin olive oil

- Spices: garlic

- Herbs: basil

- Fish: salmon

- Seafood: shrimp

- Poultry: chicken

- Dairy: yogurt

- Eggs: eggs

- Wine: red wine (optional)

- Are there any foods that I should avoid on the Mediterranean diet?

- The Mediterranean diet does not ban any foods completely

How can I incorporate the Mediterranean diet into my daily routine?

You can make small changes like switching from whatever fats you use now to extra virgin olive oil, eating a handful of raw nuts every day as a healthy replacement for processed snacks, adding whole-grain bread or other whole grains to the meal, beginning or ending each meal with a salad, adding more and different vegetables to the menu, eating at least three servings a week of legumes, and eating less meat.

Please note that these answers are general in nature, and individual dietary needs may vary based on your specific health condition, stage of disease, and other factors. Always consult with a healthcare professional for personalized advice.

# CONCLUSION

The beauty of the Mediterranean diet is when you make it a habit that will last you a lifetime, Here are some ways to make the Mediterranean diet a lifelong habit and enjoy its benefits:

1. Substitute unhealthy fats with healthy ones: Start by substituting most of your butter for a small amount of olive oil. Olive oil is the principal source of fat in the Mediterranean diet.

2. Eat more plant-based foods: Make vegetables the hero of your dish. Fill your plate with less meat and more vegetables. Go meatless at least once a week. The Mediterranean diet encourages consuming unlimited vegetables and fruits, along with whole grains, lean proteins, healthy fats, and limiting red meat and sugar.

3. Include more legumes and fish in your diet: Cook more meals with beans. Enjoy fish and seafood twice a week. Oily fish like salmon, mackerel, and sardines are good for your heart and brain.

4. Replace unhealthy snacks with healthy ones: Eat a handful of raw nuts every day as a healthy replacement for processed snacks.

5. Stay hydrated: Substitute most of your soda for water.

6. Enjoy fresh fruits daily: Substitute a daily dessert for daily fresh fruit.

7. Focus on overall eating patterns rather than strict formulas and calculations.

Here are more ways to make the Mediterranean diet a lifelong habit:

1. Switch to Extra Virgin Olive Oil: Switch from whatever fats you use now to extra virgin olive oil.

2. Eat Nuts and Olives: Include these in your daily diet.

3. Add Whole Grains: Add whole-grain bread or other whole grains to your meals.

4. Begin or End Each Meal with a Salad: This can help increase your intake of vegetables.

5. Add More and Different Vegetables to the Menu: Variety can make your meals more interesting and enjoyable.

6. Eat Legumes Three Times a Week: Options include lentils, chickpeas, beans, and peas.

7. Eat Less Meat: Choose lean poultry in moderate, 3- to 4-ounce portions. Save red meat for occasional consumption or use meat as a condiment, accompanied by lots of vegetables, as in stews, stir-fries, and soups.

8. Eat More Fish: Aim for two to three servings a week.

9. Substitute Wine in Moderation for Other Alcoholic Beverages.